Red Light Therapy

The Essential Guide Of The Miracle Near And Infra-Red Light For Fat Loss, Anti-aging, Muscle Gain And Brain Improvement

Judith C. Taylor

Bluesource And Friends

This book is brought to you by Bluesource And Friends, a happy book publishing company.

Our motto is **"Happiness Within Pages"**
We promise to deliver amazing value to readers with our books.
We also appreciate honest book reviews from our readers.

Connect with us on our Facebook page
www.facebook.com/bluesourceandfriends and stay tuned to our latest book promotions and free giveaways.

Don't forget to claim your **FREE** books!

Brain Teasers:

https://tinyurl.com/karenbrainteasers

Harry Potter Trivia:

https://tinyurl.com/wizardworldtrivia

Sherlock Puzzle Book (Volume 2)

https://tinyurl.com/Sherlockpuzzlebook2

Also check out our other books
"67 Lateral Thinking Puzzles"

https://tinyurl.com/thinkingandriddles

"Rookstorm Online Saga"

https://tinyurl.com/rookstorm

"Korman's Prayer"

https://tinyurl.com/kormanprayer

"The Convergence"

https://tinyurl.com/bloodcavefiction

"The Hardest Sudokos In Existence

(Ranked As The Hardest Sudoku Collection

Available In The Western World)"

https://tinyurl.com/MasakiSudoku

Introduction

Congratulations on getting *Red Light Therapy"*, and thank you for doing so.

The following chapters will discuss all that you need to know when it comes to working with red light therapy. There are a lot of different disorders and diseases that are common in our world. And, for the most part, we rely on harmful medications and expensive surgeries to help us deal with them. The problem is that these treatments are often worse than the actual condition, causing us to ruin our health in the process. Being able to find a treatment method that repairs the cells in a natural manner and also helps us to really take care of our bodies and get the most out of it, without a lot of bad side effects in the process, is so critical. But where are we going to find this?

This is where red light therapy comes into play. The light is able to get into our bodies and repair some of the parts of the cells that are damaged or even cancerous. By changing up some of the enzymes in the cells, and getting rid of the "bad stuff" that should not be there, red light therapy can allow us to clear out the body and get it back to good working order. And, all of this can be done with no negative side effects!

This guidebook is going to spend some time looking at the basics of red light therapy. In the first section, we are going to dive into some of the science behind the therapy and how it works. We will look at the therapy, what it does to the cells, the conditions in which it is able to clear up and help, and how it is going to be able to heal us in a natural and healthy manner. We will even discuss how this treatment is able to clear up cancer and other bad cells in the body!

Once we have a better understanding of how this treatment works, and some of the science and studies that come with it, it is time to move on to actually using the treatment. The second section of this guidebook will discuss some of the steps you can take to do an effective treatment with red light therapy, even on your own at home. It also touches upon some of the common mistakes to avoid, tips to get the most out of it, and even a few success stories to show just how successful this treatment can be.

There are alot of treatments out there that promise to be the best when it comes to the many health concerns that people deal with. But a lot of them are going to be dangerous, invasive, and, in some cases, even fatal. When you choose to use red light therapy, you can heal your body in a manner that is healthy and natural, without all of the bad; just the good. When you are ready to learn more about red light therapy and what it can do for your life, make sure to turn over the page of this guidebook to help you get started!

There are plenty of books on this subject on the market, so thanks again for choosing this one! Every effort was made to ensure it is full of as much useful information as possible. Please, enjoy!

Part 1: The Science Behind Red Light Therapy

Chapter 1: What Conditions Can Light Therapy Help With?

When we hear that something as simple as light therapy is able to make us feel better, and is able to ensure that we are going to be able to fight off a lot of disorders and diseases, we think that it sounds strange. We may not believe someone who tells us that this is true. And we may be worried about whether this works, or if it is something that is made up!

The good news is that, over the past 100 years, both red light and infrared light therapies have been studied extensively. Studies have been done on many different animals, but also on humans, to see what effects these therapies are going to make. And since a lot of the cellular metabolic processes for humans as well as other creatures are similar, the benefits to the health of these therapies are going to be similar too.

There are a lot of different diseases and conditions that can be improved with the help of these therapies, and some studies are going to show more of them as time goes on. A few of these studies have been established well, thanks to meta-analysis and scientific reviews. But remember that there are some studies on these topics that are more controversial, and may need a bit more research before we are able to prove that it is true.

Some of the different conditions that can allow you to see relief and make you feel better when you use light therapy include:

1. Acne
2. Addiction
3. Alzheimer's
4. Bell's Palsy
5. Bone fractures
6. Burn Scars
7. COPD

8. Glaucoma

9. Hypothyroidism

10. Hand, foot and mouth disease

11. Obesity

12. Muscle pain

13. Neck pain

14. Stroke

15. Skin aging

16. Osteoporosis

17. Different types of arthritis

18. Traumatic brain injury

19. Testosterone deficiency

20. Wound healing

And these are just a few of the benefits out there! There are a ton more, and it is believed that, on some level or another, you will be able to use red light therapy in order to help improve your health and make you feel better. Despite the huge number of scientific papers that have been published on this kind of therapy, there are still things that we still don't understand when it comes to light therapy, and this is why many researchers are still completing therapies in order to figure out what else they can be used for.

Chapter 2: The Top Benefits of Red Light Therapy

As we are learning more and more over time, there are a lot of different benefits that come with using this kind of therapy, and it is going to be able to permeate throughout our whole body to make us feel better and improve our health. But there are a few benefits that you are going to find that are going to be at the top when most people choose to give red light therapy, or other light therapies, a try. Some of the benefits that come with red light therapy include:

Melts the Belly Fat

According to the Center for Disease Control, 26.5 percent of adults in the United States are considered obese. Those who are obese have an increased risk of a lot of different conditions that are hard on their health, including cancer, type-2 diabetes, stroke, and heart disease. Plus, the medical costs for conditions associated with being obese will be high until the weight goes down.

There are a ton of different programs out there that promise to help you lose weight, but you may find that working with red light therapy could be the answer that you need. In 2015, a team of researchers from the Federal University of Sao Paulo in Brazil tested what would happen with light therapy on 64 participants. They were set up into two groups: One had exercise along with phototherapy, and the other one had just the exercise without the phototherapy. It took place over 20 weeks, and participants would need to work out three times a week.

During this, at the end of a workout program, one participant group was going to get light therapy, while the other would not. What was interesting was that women who got light therapy after exercise would double up the amount of fat that they lost during this time period, as compared to just exercising alone. Adding to this, participants who received red light therapy found that they had an increased skeletal muscle mass as compared to the other group.

An Increase in Bone Density

Bone density, which is the ability of the body to build up new bones over time, is so important when one is trying to recover from any injuries. It can also be an important issue for the elderly, as our bones start to become weaker with age. But it may be possible to work with red light in order to help increase our bone density. In fact, there have been a few studies that have taken a look at this, including:

1. 2003: One study concluded that LLIT had a positive effect on the repair of bone defects that were implanted with inorganic bovine bone.

2. 2006: Another study concluded that the results of their study, along with others, showed that bones irradiated mostly with infrared wavelengths through several factors like bone neo-formation and collagen deposition, especially when compared to bones that did not receive light therapy at the time.

3. 2008: A final study concluded that using laser technology has been able to improve the clinical results of bone surgeries. It helped to improve the results of any surgery on the bone and helped to promote more comfort after the operation while also promoting quicker healing.

These studies show us that, not only are we going to see some benefits when it comes to our bones, through making them stronger with the light therapy, but it can also help us after we suffer from a break or other injury to the bone. It can even help us after surgery by increasing the speed of recovery and by easing our recovery process.

Enhances Brain Function

Nootropics have seen a big spike in popularity throughout the years, and there are a lot of people who are using these kinds of drugs to help them enhance the functioning of their brain in terms of motivation, creativity, and memory. The positive effects that we are able to see with red light are shown in many studies, and can be even more powerful and safe overall as compared to using nootropic drugs.

In fact, according to researchers from the University of Texas, it was possible to put these infrared laser lights near the forehead of healthy volunteers. A study was conducted, and they measured how this affected the cognitive parameters of the individuals. Those who were treated saw improvements in their memory, reaction time, and also an increase in their positive emotional state when they came in for a two-week follow up period after the treatment.

This research shows us that this therapy can be a non-invasive treatment to increase brain functions related to the emotional and cognitive dimensions.

Increases Your Levels of Testosterone

Throughout history, the essence of a man has been linked back to the primarily male hormone that is known as "testosterone". At around the age of 30, most men find that the levels of their testosterone have started to decline, and this would mean that they will see some negative changes in their mental and physical health. This lower production of testosterone will result in a reduced amount of sexual function, reduced muscle mass, lower energy levels, and even an increased amount of fat in the body, just to name some of the issues that could come up.

When you add this in with the idea that there are so many environmental contaminants, stress, and poor nutrition that plague many men throughout the world today, it really isn't a surprise that this low testosterone level is becoming an epidemic.

In 2013, a group of Korean researchers studied what would happen when infrared laser light was put to the testicular region in men. The 30 male rats were split up into three groups: There was one control group, and then the two other groups were exposed to either near infrared light or red light. This was done for five days.

When the trial was done, the rats which were not treated did not see any kind of increase in testosterone levels. The rats which were given one-half hour treatment of light therapy each day saw that their testosterone levels were elevated. The group that had the near infrared light saw their Serum T levels increase by a significant amount. And the group that was administered red light therapy saw pretty much the same increase in the process.

This means that, if men are dealing with low levels of testosterone and some other health problems that come with it, it may be possible to benefit from red light therapy. With the help of this therapy, it is possible for you to increase your levels of testosterone while, in the meantime, reducing some of the different health issues that come with this condition.

Can Help You to Eliminate Depression and Anxiety

Depression and anxiety are big issues that many millions of people throughout the world are dealing with on a daily basis. In fact, it is believed that 121 million people throughout the world are suffering from depression, and this is only for the number of people who are officially diagnosed with the disorder. In addition, it is found that there are at least 40 million adults older than 18, in just the United States alone, who are dealing with anxiety. These two problems are out there, but the treatments for them are often ineffective, toxic, or can, at best, numb one out, and at worst, can make one sick and cause a lot of health problems.

This is why there is some special interest when it comes to working with red light therapy to see if anxiety and depression can both be solved with the help of this therapy. We will start by taking a look at depression first.

In 2009, a group of researchers from Harvard University tested infrared lights on 10 subjects with major depression. Researchers applied the light right on the forehead on the patients for one session that lasted 16 minutes. After one treatment of this therapy, the patients experienced a highly significant reduction in both anxiety and depression, with the greatest reduction showing up over a two-week period.

What this means is that the near-infrared light therapy resulted in a long-lasting reduction for both anxiety and depression. And this happens with just one treatment. Imagine what can happen when you do this on a regular basis to help with anxiety and depression!

Relieves Pain

According to a study in 2015 done by the National Institute of Health, America is a nation of pain. This is because nearly 50 million American adults reported that they had been going through some kind of pain daily for the three months previous. Some of the most common pain medication that people are going to reach for when they deal with pain includes options like Ibuprofen or Tylenol. Interestingly, these are all linked to heart attacks, cancer, and strokes. Except for aspirin, which is able to reduce the risks in some cases, these NSAIDS (Non-Steroidal Anti-Inflammatory Drugs) could be dangerous for your health.

Basically, even though we feel better when we take these medications, we are giving ourselves something that can ruin our health. But with the help of infrared light therapy, we could reduce pain without needing any medication at all!

Heals Arthritis

Another benefit that comes with using red light therapy is that it is able to help heal arthritis. Arthritis is a crippling ailment that many people throughout the world suffer from. In fact, between 2013 and 2015, it is believed that almost 23 percent of adults in the United States were diagnosed with some form of arthritis. This means that a good 55 million people will benefit from using something like light therapy to help them.

A Harvard professor from the Department of Dermatology, Dr. Michael R. Hamblin, published a study in 2013 to see how red light therapy would be able to help with arthritis in patients. After inducing arthritis in rats and then treating them with just one treatment of red light therapy, their inflammation reduced quite a bit in just one day. This could be great news for those who are dealing with arthritis and would like to get a break from some of the pain.

Other Benefits of Red Light Therapy

We have spent a lot of time in this chapter, looking at some of the different ways that this therapy will be able to improve our health and make things better. But there are so many more options that are going to come into play that will make this kind of therapy worth your time. We are going to take a look at a few of them now.

First, this treatment is going to help with rejuvenating the skin. The red light is going to be able to penetrate under the skin to help bring more blood to the surface, and it can boost your blood circulation. This therapy is also going to help increase the production of collagen and elastin of the skin. The overall effect to this is a repair to the damaged cells that may be there, giving the skin the appearance of being youthful again. This means that the red light is going to be a great treatment for removing some of the blemishes that you have, tightening the skin, and repairing some damaged cells.

Next on the list is pain relief. This kind of therapy is not only going to improve the appearance of the skin, but is also a great treatment to rely on when you need some relief from pain. Because this therapy is able to penetrate deep into the body, it is going to be able to repair some components of the cells as well. And it is going to have an added benefit of being able to increase the production of endorphins in the body and can help block some transmitters that cause us pain.

The third benefit is that red light therapy can help to rehabilitate injuries, and there are some professional athletes who will swear by how this kind of therapy can help them to get back into the game and be healed from the injuries.

The reason that this kind of therapy is so efficient in increasing recovery time is due to the fact that this kind of light stimulates ATP production. This chemical is able to reduce the inflammation and swelling that is found in the body, while increasing white blood cells, which can help to repair any of the tissue that has been damaged, no matter where it has occurred within the body.

And finally, one reason that a lot of people like to work with red light therapy is that it can help to reduce or eliminate acne throughout the body. The red light is able to reach into your skin and then activate the hemoglobin that is there. This is going to limit the amount of blood supply to your sebaceous glands that cause acne, making it harder for them to do the work that they need. This will prevent the skin cells from getting too oily and producing acne. For those who are dealing with acne and none of the other treatments seem to be working, red light therapy may be the option that you want to work with.

As you can see, there are a lot of different health conditions that can be healed with the help of red light therapy. And as more people decide to try it out, and more studies are done on how this light works and how it can affect your body and health, you will find that, likely, we will be able to link this red light therapy to a lot of other health conditions. You may find that, out of the options listed above, red light therapy is going to be able to help you with some of your conditions.

Chapter 3: Red Light Therapy and Cancer

It is important to take a look at red light therapy and how it may be possible to use it to help us deal with and fight off cancer. As we go through this guidebook and study how the red light works, and how it is able to affect the cells and all the different parts in our body, we will start to understand how it can be used to treat many diseases out there, including cancer. But first, we need to explore a bit about cancer and how this disease works. It may be different than what we are used to hearing or thinking about this horrible disease.

The Epidemic of Cancer

Governments throughout the world often tell us that 50 percent of people who are alive right now will develop some form of cancer in their lifetime. What is the most frightening about this is that, if we are diagnosed with this disease, then the treatments that are often recommended to us can be a problem as well. Think back to a time when someone you knew had to go through radiotherapy, chemotherapy, or even surgery to help with cancer. And, often, they come out of these treatments looking and feeling much worse than they did before.

Of course, just by reading up on what these various treatments should tell us that they are bad. Cutting someone open, adding some poison to their bodies, and even burning them with some of the radiation that is also found in a nuclear bomb is, of course, going to make their health worse than before. Our own experiences as humans can validate this over and over again, and it may be time to consider a different cure when we look to cancer, rather than using things that may work, but end up actually harming the health of the individual.

According to Dr. Hardin B Jones, a professor of medical physics at the University of California, Berkley, "My studies have proved conclusively that untreated cancer victims live up to four times longer than treated individuals. If one has cancer and opts to do nothing at all, he will live longer and feel better than if he undergoes radiation, chemotherapy, or surgery, other than when used in immediate life-threatening situations."

Most of us would not take it this far. In fact, we know that treating cancer is important and we want to be able to do something about it, whether we are the ones dealing with cancer or someone we love is dealing with cancer. The problem is that many of the current treatments out there are not cutting it. They sometimes work, but the negative consequences that come with it just makes it really hard to be worth putting yourself through that kind of turmoil and ill health.

The Metabolic Disease of Cancer

One of the largest myths out there and that has been taught to us by the cancer industry is that the cancer cell is like a microscopic terrorist that has one job, and one job only – to kill the person. The idea that cancer is only going to kill us if we don't go in and do something drastic to kill it first is pure myth, and that is part of the problem.

There is no scientific evidence that has suggested that cancer cells or tumors are actually going to cause that much harm to the individual, even though we all tense up in fear and worry when we hear the word "cancer". In addition, *The Cancer Genome Atlas Project*, started in 2005 by The National Cancer Institute, was deemed as a failure. There was not a single gene mutation or even a combination of mutations that came together, that was found to be absolutely responsible for starting the disease of cancer.

This may seem shocking, but it is basically because cancer is not seen as a genetic disease. It has been almost 100 years since Dr. Otto Warburg, a Nobel Prize Winning scientist, discovered that a cancer cell was just a regular cell, like the millions of others found in our body, which had the mitochondria damaged in some manner.

The mitochondria are the tiny particles found within the cells that are responsible for producing energy for that cell. So, when we are talking about what we typically see as a cancer cell, we are just looking at a cell that is defective metabolically, or a cell that is inured and is in need of some repair to help it get better.

After *The Cancer Genome Atlas Project* proved to us that cancer is not really a genetic disease, but more of a metabolic one, James Watson, known as the father of DNA, recommended that we need to shift our focus in research over cancer away from the world of genetics, because it is not the major problem that we are dealing with. Instead, we need to move the focus to metabolic processes and how we can fix cancer that way.

Having a good understanding of some of the basics of metabolism of cells and how we can use this information to repair metabolic defects can empower someone to find ways to enhance the natural healing process of the body, without drugs or any of the bad treatments that are usually offered for cancer. This ensures that we are better equipped to handle cancer and see results without harming our health in the process.

And there are many who believe that infrared light therapy is one of the treatments introduced later on to help with this. It gives you a chance to use something that is natural to heal the root cause of cancer and even prevent its occurrence in the first place. This may be an idea that seems crazy to a lot of people, and some may struggle with trying to move away from the traditional forms of taking care of the body. But isn't it kind of crazy that we rely on such harmful treatments to deal with cancer, including: Radiation, chemotherapy, and even surgery, rather than methods that are more natural and good for us?

Chapter 4: How Does Red Light Heal?

Now it is time to take a look at how this red light is going to be able to work to your benefit in helping to heal the body: Trillions of cells that make up who we are will find small structures inside of them known as "mitochondria". These are responsible for the cell's energy production, in a process called "metabolism".

When a cell is given the nutrients and more than it needs in order to properly metabolize, a process that is going to involve some chemical oxidation of glucose over into carbon dioxide into the mitochondria, this is a sign that the cell is healthy and doing what it is supposed to. If the breakdown of metabolism within the cells starts to happen, then this is when we start to see more disease and cancer throughout the body.

It is true that almost all of the main diseases we see in humans have been linked back to the mitochondrial activity in our cells. Understanding which foods, as well as what other factors are able to enhance metabolism, and which are going to inhibit this metabolism, can be a lifesaver because it can help you to not only prevent the diseases that are going on in your body, but can even reverse some that you are already suffering from.

When you go through the process of red light therapy, the skin is going to be exposed to a laser of a really low level. You will do this for a few times a week for a certain treatment time based on your needs. You can do this indefinitely, but most people are going to pick to do this for a certain kind of condition, and the treatment will last for one to two months until that condition is dealt with fully.

You are able to use a red light therapy device from your own home if you choose, but there are also a lot

41

of professionals who work in cosmetic clinics and other similar places that will be able to do this treatment for you as well. Either way, as long as the right devices are being used, you will see that red light therapy will be a great way to improve your health.

For those who believe in the power of red light therapy, believe that the low level of the laser will help to kick start the ability of the body to recover from a variety of conditions, diseases, and more. In addition, this laser will help the body increase the production of collagen, increase blood flow, and repair your tissues.

Now, we need to take some time to look at the mechanics of how this kind of therapy is going to work. The way that this works will be similar to what we see with other laser treatments, but the red light is going to work with a lower wavelength. This allows us to use it on areas that are a bit more sensitive, including the skin and the eyes, while still being safe.

When we are able to expose the skin to this light energy, it is going to release more of a chemical that is known as ATP, or adenosine triphosphate, which is believed to help the body work to form some new capillaries, boost collagen production, and repair some of the tissues that have been damaged in the body.

For these reasons, there are a lot of times that people will choose to use red light therapy to help themselves. It has been used to help with: Treating issues in arthritis, heal burns, and smooth out stretch marks. These are just a few of the different ways that you are able to work with the therapy, and we have discussed a few of them, along with the research that backs it up, earlier in this guidebook.

The neat thing about this is that the first FDA-approved use for this kind of therapy and the device that comes with it was one that was used to help speed up wound healing that was going slowly. The way that this was done is that the laser of red light would penetrate the skin between 8 and 10 millimeters, and this helped it to later be absorbed deeper into the body. Over time, when this was used properly, it helped affect the immune system, metabolic processes, and the nervous system, to name a few.

This brings us to the point of how red light therapy is different from some of the other therapy types that are out there. To keep it simple, it is all going to come down to the wavelengths of the red light. This treatment is going to emit some red light that is visible, and the lasers are going to be emitted at 60 nm. Some of these treatments are going to use more of a near-infrared light above 700 nm, or below visible red light, which would be closer to 590 nm. And then there are some devices that are going to combine blue and red light together. It all depends on the type of light that you decide to purchase.

When we compare this to what is seen with traditional laser therapy, we will find that these treatments are going to emit light at a higher density than red light therapy. This causes more damage to the tissues of the body and can cause destruction or more if you are not careful. This is not a potential problem with red light therapy, because of the very low level laser that is emitted.

The goal of traditional laser therapy is to damage the skin because this is believed to promote body healing and revitalizing faster than it would without the treatment. Red light therapy is not going to have enough power or heat to do this, and you don't have to worry about it burning, destroying or injuring the tissues of the body. This is why it is seen as a more efficient method for healing than others.

It will work in a manner similar to some of the other laser therapies out there, in that the laser that is emitted from the light is going to be able to help heal the body and repair some of the cells that are in the body. But it is not going to come with any of the potential danger like we see with other methods, which makes it so much better to work with.

Lowering the Metabolism with Some Environmental Toxins

One thing we need to focus on and understand when it comes to cellular metabolism is that, all the steps that we will work with are going to be catalyzed thanks to one specific enzyme. This enzyme is known as "cytochrome c oxidase". This enzyme was discovered by Dr. Otto Warburg in 1926.

So, why do we need to be able to understand this particular enzyme? This enzyme is responsible for the oxygen that is used by the cells, in that it can interact directly with that oxygen, and will catalyze the very last step in the process of metabolism. This is very important if we want to make sure that the metabolism of the cells is going to be done in a proper manner.

Through his research, Dr. Warburg found that, when we are able to inhibit this enzyme, we would end up taking a cell that was previously healthy and then turn it cancerous. And this information has been validated through the years with other studies and experiments.

This is a huge finding that we need to spend more time on. When one enzyme is taken out, harmed, or inhibited in some manner, then this is going to be a bad thing for you. It means that the body is going to struggle with doing the metabolism that it needs, and this causes the cell to go from one that is healthy to one that has issues and could be considered cancerous overall. According to scientists from the University of Pennsylvania in 2015, "Defects in cytochrome c oxidase expression induce a metabolic shift to glycolysis and carcinogenesis."

This supports what we have been talking about all along: When the cells do not have this particular enzyme, or there is some other reason why this enzyme is not doing the work that it should, then there would be some issues along the way. The cells are going to deal with health conditions of all kinds, cancer, and more. Ensuring that this enzyme is able to work in the manner that it should, and learning how to make the metabolism work properly will make a difference in the overall health of the body.

There have actually been a few toxins that are going to inhibit the activity of this enzyme, including: Unsaturated fatty acids, X-ray radiation, EVB radiation, serotonin, estrogen, aluminum phosphide, carbon dioxide, cyanide, chemotherapy, and more. You can control a few of these on your own if you would like, such as the fatty acids that you are eating, but there are a few that are a bit harder to control.

Let's take a look at how these are going to work: When you are exposed in some manner to any of the above contaminants of the environment, the cells are going to produce a free radical that is known as "nitric oxide". This free radical is going to bind directly to the cytochrome c oxidase that we need so desperately, and it will end up deactivating it at some point. As long as the nitric oxide stays bound to the enzyme, it means that the cell is not able to metabolize in the manner that it should, giving it a defective cancer metabolism in the process.

How to Enhance the Metabolism of the Cell with Some Red Light

Now, we need to take a look at what red light therapy is going to be able to do in order to help us out. The impact that we are going to see with near infrared and red light on the metabolism of our cells is really unique. It has spurred a lot of studies throughout the years. In fact, both of these lights have been shown to

49

actually unbind the nitric oxide from the cytochrome c oxidase enzyme from cells.

When the red light is able to remove the nitric oxide, it is going to do some things that are amazing. The cytochrome c oxidase is able to get back to work, and it is going to be more energized. This helps to supercharge the activity of the enzyme, speed up the metabolism that is there, and will ensure that the cell gets back to its old healthy self rather than being diseased and even cancerous, causing trouble for you.

This is good news for you because it means that you are going to see an enhancement in how the cells are able to metabolize again. They are going to get back to what they should do naturally, which some kind of environmental toxins has stopped them with. When this happens, it means that you are going to be able to enjoy a bunch of beneficial physiological effects that are going to emerge when the metabolic activity increases. Some of these beneficial effects include:

1. A reduction in the number of free radicals found in the cells.

2. A reduction in the amount of inflammation found in the body, and the negative effects of the health when the inflammation goes down.

3. A reduction in the amount of lactic acid that builds up.

4. A reduction in the number of stress hormones found in the body, which everyone is going to be able to benefit from.

5. An increased amount of CO_2 production.

6. An increased amount of blood that will flow through the body, helping us to clean out the body easier, get more energy, and just improve our health overall.

7. An increase in the amount of cellular oxygenation.

8. An increase in the amount of energy ATP production throughout the body as well.

As you can see here, there are already a lot of health benefits that you will reap when you work with the red light therapy and other types of light therapy in the process. This is going to be important because we will be able to improve so much with these lights allowing our bodies to heal in a more natural manner.

We could choose to take a lot of medications to do this, but that will just mask the problem and hide the symptoms, rather than give us the actual relief that we want. The second we stop taking the medications is the second we are going to start feeling sick again. But with something like red light therapy, which takes care of the condition and helps the body to heal naturally, you will feel relief faster, and you will enjoy better health in no time. And this can make a world of difference to so many people.

It is all these beneficial physiological options above that are going to account for most, if not all, of the different effects that people are going to benefit from when they use near-infrared or red light therapies to improve their health. Think about all of the health benefits that we have talked about already in this guidebook, along with so many more that are yet to be discovered, and you can see why this light is so powerful, especially when it comes to metabolism in the cells.

To help us summarize this, both the infrared and the red light are able to penetrate deeply into the tissues that are in your body. This is so important because they are then going to help reduce the amount of nitric acid in our body. This healing power of removing the nitric acid and making it disappear allows the cells to finally heal and do the work that they are meant to. With just a few sessions with this light therapy, you can get relief and turn cells that could be cancerous back into healthy and happy cells again.

Chapter 5: Is Red Light Therapy Actually Safe to Use?

The next question that many people are going to have when it comes to working with red light therapy is whether it is safe to use or not. There is some worry that this is going to be strange, or that it will be so strong that something can go wrong. When we look at all of the things that it is able to do, it is easy to see why there could be some worries about the safety of using this therapy.

The thing to remember here is that this is not some strange method that is going to shock you or something powerful that you need to be worried about. This is using light. Just like the light from the sun that can help to improve your mood because it provides you with vitamin D, red light therapy is going to be just light that comes in at a frequency that helps you get a lot of health benefits. It is as simple as that!

Unlike a lot of the different surgical treatments or drug treatments that are offered in the medical world today, red light therapy is safe and low on side effects. Many surgeries and medications come with a huge list of side effects that are at least adverse if not fatal in some cases.

We have all seen those commercials that go through and list out all of the negative side effects that come with the medications that are recommended. They promise to give you some great results, but then you have to worry about the bad side effects. And in some cases, these side effects are going to be so bad, it is easy to wonder if it is worth your time to take the medication or just live with the disease or the pain.

But with red light therapy, you will find that there are very few adverse side effects, and most people experience nothing bad at all. In fact, when compared to some of the other methods out there, red light therapy is seen as one of the most effective, as well as one of the safest, of all the treatments.

According to Dr. Michael Hamblin, who is a professor and scientist from Harvard, "In terms of side effects, there are very few side effects. I've occasionally heard of people who put light on their head – I think one person had a headache and a few people felt excessively sleepy."

These side effects are hardly anything to worry about. You may have a slight headache as you adjust to the detoxification, etc., of working with the light therapy, and you may need to take a nap when the therapy is done if it makes you a bit sleepy, but that is it! And this is out of hundreds of studies and research done on lots of participants, and most didn't experience them at all.

You may not have time to read through all the different abstracts on the studies that have been done on red light therapies, but with the research in this guidebook and with other books as well, you will find that there are like no adverse side effects in most of the patients who went through these studies.

One of the reasons that you will not read about a bunch of people doing red light therapy and experiencing negative side effects is that the intensity of the energy from the red light wavelengths will be really low. The amount of exposure that you are going to get from the energy of the red light is going to be so low that your tissue temperature is only going to increase by about a tenth of a degree overall.

This is hardly any rise in temperature, and that is going to be great news. It is never going to cause any kind of burns or thermal injury to the body, so you are able to use the light therapy even over long periods of time, and not have to worry about any injuries to the body due to the light.

You will also find that the devices that you use for near infrared and red light therapy are going to emit a small amount of light. In fact, most of the time, the device will emit as low as 12 watts of light. Even with this low amount (a lightbulb for your home lighting is often going to be 70 watts or more), you are going to see that there are some remarkably potent effects on the body.

As just discussed, you will find that, because this kind of therapy is going to have pretty much no thermal effects on the body, it is a great option to use when you have a fresh injury that you want to work on healing. These injuries are going to be more sensitive to heat, so you do not want to work with therapies that rely on heat.

Instead, they need some kind of therapy that is low on heat. The higher heat is just going to irritate the injury, and could even make the inflammation and the swelling harder to work with and alot worse. These heat sources could make the pain worse in the process. But with red light therapy, you will find that, since there is no worry about heat, it is safe to use even on these heat-sensitive injuries.

And finally, if you are still worried that red light therapy is not safe to use, it is actually an FDA-approved therapy for a couple of different health conditions, and the US Government considers this kind of therapy as safe for most people.

While it is still a good idea to talk to your doctor before you decide to rely solely on red light therapy for your treatment needs, it is generally seen as safe. It can work with a variety of different health conditions, and it is going to help you to see some great results in the process. And since it is easy to use, you are sure to be able to find a practitioner in your area who knows how to use the therapy, who can answer your questions about the therapy, and who can help you to go through your first (or hundredth), red light therapy treatment.

Part 2: Using the Red Light Therapy

Chapter 6: Creating Space for the Treatment

Now that we know a little bit more about red light therapy and why it is such a great treatment for different health conditions, it is time to learn some of the steps that you can take in order to really get the most out of the therapy.

In this section, we are going to talk about the five things that you need to consider when you are ready to do your own red light therapy. This includes: Finding the right space for doing the treatment, the right body position, the position of the light, the number of times that you should do the sessions, and how long the sessions should last.

One thing to remember before we start with the first part is that simplicity is key. This treatment is meant to make your life a bit easier. It is not meant to make you feel like there are a lot of particulars to remember, and you should not feel like you have to second guess yourself all of the time. The one rule to remember and that you want to follow is that you need to make things as simple as possible. This helps to make the therapy sessions more efficient and enjoyable.

So now that we have that out of the way, it is time to look at how you can create a good space to do these treatments. Think of it this way: If you had to start out each session by carrying the device up three flights of stairs, then plug it in and lay down on a cold hard cement floor for fifteen minutes or more, how likely would you be to keep doing the treatment, even if it did provide results?

Hopefully, the space that you pick out for doing the therapy is not this bad, but it is a good illustration of what you can do so as to see the importance of working with a designated space for the purpose of therapy. If you are not able to make these sessions as pleasurable and simple as possible, then, most likely, you are not going to stick with doing the sessions for any length of time. And the more work you have to do and the more uncomfortable these sessions are, the more likely that you will only do the treatment for a few times before giving up in exasperation.

This is why it is such a good idea to create some place in your office or home that is dedicated to this light therapy treatment. In fact, it is going to be essential for you to get the best results when you are working with this session. And the space that you pick needs to make the treatment itself as simple and as pleasurable as you possibly can.

Now, you will be able to set this up in any manner that you would like. You may find that working with a yoga mat, a blanket, or even a towel spread out on the floor where you need to lay or sit down on can make it more comfortable. Adding a pillow or two can be great as well. And, some people find that it is best if you are able to lay on a bed or a cot to add in a bit more comfort to the situation.

In addition to the above options for comfort, you may decide to keep a timer in place. Some patients like to just use the timer on their phone for this, which is fine. But if you want to work with a designated timer just for the red light therapy, then make sure that you leave it in the treatment space. This saves time and effort from always having to look for it later.

Another consideration when picking out a space for your treatments is that there should be some power outlet nearby. Your light device has to stay plugged in at all times during the therapy, and if it can recharge in between sessions, this can make things a bit easier.

From there, you may think about what else you would like to have in your treatment space. This is your special space, and it is hopefully going to be set up in a manner that will help you relax and stay focused during the session. Each person is going to bring in different things to the mix, and this is fine. But you may want to consider what would make you the most comfortable and relaxed, and what will help you gain the right focus when you are working through light therapy.

With the space in mind, also consider when you would like to do the light therapy. It is often recommended that you do it either in the morning or in the evening. You can choose the time period that works best for you. Both of these are beneficial times, and you have to go with one that is either going to help energize you for the morning, or give you some repair in the evening after a hard day.

For example, some people find that doing therapy in the morning is best for them. The red light therapy is going to help you to be more energized and ready for the day. It can add more focus, improve memory, and can repair the cells and helps you to detoxify your body before you get out for the day. Depending on the kind of condition that you are dealing with, you may find that the morning treatment timing is going to be more efficient for you in the process.

But then there are also some benefits that come with doing the light treatments in the evening. This is a good way to repair any of the damage that happened to your cells during the day and can relieve some of the headaches, stress, and more that have built up throughout your daily life. This one works well if you are suffering from stress and other conditions that make it hard for you to fall asleep at night.

The main point of this section is that we need to have a good space for treatment and choose the time that works best for us. Your goal, if you have the room to make it happen, is to have a designated space that is just for this therapy, but try to at least get something that is going to be comfortable and will allow you to focus and relax while the red light therapy is doing its work.

Chapter 7: The Body Position During the Red Light Therapy

In the last chapter, we took some time looking at the best places to set up your treatments in order to help you be relaxed, comfortable, and focused on the session. Now we are going to move on to the second part of this, which is the body position. The way that you are going to position the body when you do one of the treatment sessions is going to matter. If you have your body placed in some kind of position in a way that is uncomfortable, and you are not able to relax all the way, then it is not going to take long before this stops holding your interest and you decide to not use the device and get its benefits any longer.

Remember that we are going to be more motivated to do things that we find pleasant and rewarding. This is why we need to make sure that we find a position for the body that is comfortable and still gives us a chance to relax all the way, or we will stop. The good news is there are three options that you are able to use when it comes to how to position your body while still getting the full benefits of the red light therapy. The three methods that you are able to use include lying down, sitting, and standing.

The Standing Body Position

There are a few devices for red light therapy that are designed to help those who plan to stand up for their whole session. These can include some LED light panels that will be held with a stand, or placed on the wall. There are also some vertical booths with a swinging door to get in and out that can help with the treatment.

While the idea of standing up for your treatment may seem like a good idea to try, do you really want to stand stuck in one place for a possible 20 minutes two times a day depending on your treatment? Standing in one spot for a long period of time can be uncomfortable because of the weight of supporting your body. And it may be really hard for you to fully relax and be as comfortable as you need to in order to see the results.

If this is what you are the most comfortable with using during the treatment, or what works the best for the space that you are in, then go ahead and use it. But for most people, it is not going to be comfortable. And you may find that standing still for that long can add in more discomfort than what you were trying to fix with the light therapy. This is why most people would prefer working with the other two body positions.

The Sitting Body Position

The second option that you are able to work with is the sitting body position. If you are able to sit in a comfortable recliner or a sofa, you are able to relax and enjoy the treatment. There are a lot of benefits of working with this because it is going to be more comfortable than standing for the treatment duration, and you get some options for where to sit.

But there are still a lot of people who are looking to go with another position because there are some disadvantages that come with this method. Some of the main downsides that come with the seated position include some of the following:

1. When you do the therapy while sitting, you need to have some supportive muscles to help you contract, preventing you from getting into full relaxation.
2. When you do the therapy while sitting, it can make it a bit harder to position the red light in the manner such that you can get a full amount of healing.

3. When you do the therapy while sitting, it is sometimes uncomfortable, and sometimes people may find it a bit painful during the therapy.

There are a lot of benefits to sitting during the therapy, and it is definitely a much better option than standing. It is a lot more comfortable to work with and can make it easier to relax and get the benefits. But, there are still some disadvantages, so you will have to compare to see if this is the method that works for you so as to reap the full benefits of the red light therapy treatment.

The Laying Down Body Position

If you are able to do this, then laying down is going to be the best option to choose. This is seen as the gold standard for red light therapy treatment sessions. Laying down is going to give you all of the comforts that you are looking for. It makes it easier to relax every single muscle in your body, and it is the only position out of the three that is the safest if you fall asleep during the treatment.

In many offices that offer this kind of therapy, the devices are going to be hung from the ceiling, with the patient lying on a massage therapy table under that light. This is one way to do it. Finding an above supportive structure that you are able to hang the light from can require some creativity, but it is something to try.

Now, this can be a bit harder to work with for some people, but if you are trying to place it on your leg, stomach or somewhere similar, it is possible to just lay it down on that area. It is not going to cause burns or any other issues, so you will be safe using it in this manner. You can then just relax as the body enjoys the red light therapy and all that it is able to provide to you.

Chapter 8: The Position of the Light During Treatment

The next thing we need to take a look at when you are doing one of our treatments is the position of the light. Since you will find that laying down is going to be the ideal position of the body when you do your treatment, most of the attention that we focus on here is going to be with where the light needs to be while you are laying down. But first, we can talk about where to put the light when you are either sitting or standing.

First, you can choose to do light therapy while standing. When standing for the treatment, the position of your light can be either on a vertical stand, or you can use a light that is mounted onto a wall near you. This is going to be beneficial because you can get the therapy without having to hold onto the light during the session. However, there is a disadvantage, in that you will have to stand up during the treatment to get the benefits.

Then, you have the choice of sitting while doing the light therapy. This is a good option, and the location for the light can be either on a table right in front of you, or you can place it on your lap facing you. The light position here is going to make it more difficult to treat any part of the body that is not the face or the chest area, since the distance is nearer for those areas when you choose this.

You can also pick some different lighting positions when you are laying down. Compared to the sitting or standing position, you will find that positioning the light for laying down is going to be easier. You can lay down in the right position, and then place the device right beside you on the floor or the bed, aiming that light at the part of the body that needs to have the treatment.

You can also choose to hang the light device from something above you if this seems like it is the best choice to use. But for most people, laying down and facing the light in the direction of the part of the body that needs the treatment, is going to be the best, and often the easiest, place to put the light.

If you need to work on pain in your lower back, you can just place the light behind you right against the area that is causing the pain and then relax. If you have a sore knee, lay down with the light against the knee. This is the same no matter what part of the body you are feeling pain or issues with, and no matter what kind of treatment you want to work with. Just lay the red light against that body part while you relax and enjoy the light that is coming in while laying down.

As we mentioned before, laying down is going to be the most ideal of the body positions when you are doing your red light therapy. It is going to afford you a lot of comforts while being safe and still making light positioning easier. It is the simplicity that you need, as we talked about before, and it ensures that you are able to relax, which is needed when you want to get the most out of the session.

Chapter 9: The Duration of the Session

The fourth thing that we need to spend some time looking through when we want to do some red light therapy is the duration of the session. This means that most people need to consider how long they want to use the red light each time they begin treatment. The amount of times that you do it during the day and the duration of the sessions is going to depend on the problem that you are trying to solve, and how bad that issue is from the beginning.

The duration of the session is going to be the number of minutes that you will expose a body part to the red light session. You may find that experimenting a bit and seeing what works the best for you is going to help you get the most efficient amount of time for each session.

There is a bit of science that has been done in order to determine the amount of time for a session to get the best results based on the condition that you are dealing with. It is also important to remember that nothing is set in stone. You may have to go for a bit longer, but then there is a chance that you will need less time in order to see results. Starting out at the base that is talked about in various studies is a good place to look at, but you can add or take away time, based on what works for you.

If you are worried about going for too long with the therapy, it is fine to start out with smaller or shorter sessions and then build up to what you want. But remember that red light therapy is going to be one of the safest therapies and treatments that you are able to do for most ailments, so there really isn't much to worry about when you go for the length of time that you have chosen for this treatment.

The first thing that you may consider doing with this treatment is to do the red light on the whole body. If you feel comfortable enough doing this, you can lie in a fetal position without any clothes on, and with the light facing a position that is right between the chest and stomach. This may sound awkward, but remember that you are alone, and that this is going to be a good way to prepare your body and get some overall healing right from the beginning.

The goal of the full body treatment is that it is going to help you to reach as many of the cells in your body as you can. From this position, if you do it the right way, you should be able to get the upper arms, the chest, the stomach, and the upper legs as well in one shot. This is great if you only have one light and you want to work on as much of your body as possible in one treatment session.

Even if you bought the light in order to help with a particular part of the body, such as your chronic pain

81

or an injured ankle, it is still a good idea to take time to work on the whole body before moving on to working with just that body part. This is one way for you to see the healing power that even a small device for red light therapy is able to do for your body.

When you decide to work with the full body treatment, you are going to notice that you feel better in no time. This is because you are working on as many of the cells in the body as possible. You may start to notice that you feel better, less depressed, and that other things are healed – things that you may not have even noticed were bothering you previously. If you decide to do this kind of treatment, you will find that working on this session for about 20 minutes is a good start.

For most people, working with the treatment for 15 to 20 minutes is enough time to get the results that you want. But you may need to experiment with this for a bit. While there is no harm with going for a bit longer on your treatment if you choose, because all it is going to do is improve your health without any negative side effects, most people like to find the timing of the session that works for them.

You can have two choices with this: You can either start with the 20 minutes for the treatment, or you can go through and slowly increase the time until you reach the one that seems to provide you with the most benefits. This one takes a bit longer, but lets you know the personalized time for the red light treatment that works the best for the disease or disorder you are dealing with.

For example, you may start out with a treatment that is five minutes long and see how that does. You may then notice that this is not long enough to provide you with all of the relief that you want, so you up to your sessions to ten minutes a day and then see how that works for you. Then you add on 15 minutes, and then 20 minutes, and so on.

You may find that you are good at 15 minutes, and don't feel like there is much of a difference between going from 15 minutes to 20 minutes. Then this means that you can pick between the two and go with the time period that is the best for you. Once you start feeling that the benefits are not getting any stronger or better when you go up in time, this is a good sign that the lowest time frame where you started feeling this way is going to be the right one for you.

In addition, you may find that each part of your body may need to have a different session duration. You may feel relief from an ankle problem after ten minutes, but find that you need closer to 20 or 25 minutes in order to help the stress or anxiety in your life. This is perfectly normal, and taking the time to experiment will make it easier to find the time frames that work best for you.

The session duration that you choose is an important consideration to think about ahead of time. Whether you choose to go with the standard timings for your condition, or you are willing to mess around a bit and see which method works the best for you, you will find that the red light therapy is going to provide you with the benefits you need. You just have to identify how long of a session you need to do to get those great benefits.

Chapter 10: The Frequency of the Sessions You Do with Red Light

Now, the fifth thing that we need to consider when we are getting ready to work with our session is the frequency of the sessions. We have to determine how often we are going to do these sessions: Whether it is a few times a day, a few times a week, or just at any time we feel the problem is flaring up again.

The session frequency will be defined as the number of treatment sessions that you are going to need to go through each day or week. As a general guideline, also considering what works for you, studies have shown that going with somewhere between two and twenty sessions per week is going to be effective. This means that you may need to get between two and three sessions a day for the treatment, although some people are just fine if they do one or two sessions spread out throughout the week.

However, you can choose the number of times that will work for you. There shouldn't be any worries about how many times you use the device, and if you want to experiment with this and use it more often than two or three times weekly, then this is fine, because red light therapy is safe and will not cause any harm with more use.

For many people at least, starting out with two treatments a day is going to work well for them. This helps to fix the cells and keeps them as healthy as possible. Over time, they may decide to go up or down on the number of sessions done based on how they are feeling. Doing one when you wake up in the morning to energize and prepare you for the day, and then doing one at night to help you get a more restful and peaceful sleep, can be the best options for your needs.

One question that is often asked here is that, since the red light is able to energize the cells inside of our bodies, do we need to worry about doing the treatment at night, and how could it interrupt the sleep of the patient? Put your mind at ease here because the answer is no, and many patients have found that doing a therapy session before they go to bed can help them to fall asleep and stay asleep better at night.

The reason for this is that the red light is going to reduce both the levels of adrenaline and cortisol in the body, which is so important to helping them to fall asleep at night. In addition, since the red light therapy is able to help us to reduce the amount of stress we are dealing with, it is even easier to fall asleep.

Of course, before you start to make some changes to what you are doing with your red light therapy treatments, take some time to try it out beforehand.

This works with all of the tips that we have looked at when it comes to the session. Figure out what position it should be in, where the light should go, how often you should do the sessions, and even the amount of times that you should do the sessions. This red light therapy treatment is meant to be something that works well for you, and taking the time to personalize it and make it fit in with your comfort level is definitely something that is important if you want to see results.

Chapter 11: Common Mistakes People Make When Using Red Light Therapy

When it comes to using red light therapy, you will find that there are a lot of great benefits that you are going to be getting: You are able to increase the density of your bones, help with weight loss, reduce anxiety and depression, learn how to reduce stress levels, and so much more. As more research is done with regard to this therapy, it is likely that almost everyone will be able to use the therapy to repair their health and make them feel so much better.

That said, it is also important to know that there are some common mistakes that you need to be careful about when you use red light therapy: You need to learn how to avoid some of these common mistakes to ensure that you are going to get the most out of your treatments, and that you will not feel like the treatment is not working for your needs or your particular health conditions. Some of the most common mistakes that beginners may make when they first decide to work with the red light therapy treatments for their health will include the following:

They Don't Do It for Long Enough

Timing your light therapy sessions is very important. If you don't spend enough time under the light each day, you may not get the full benefits that you are looking for. This is why it is important to experiment a bit and figure out how long the red light works best for your condition. Some people may be able to do ten minutes a few times a day, and others will need closer to 20 or more minutes to get the same results. Each person is going to be different, and it will really be determined by how your body responds to the light.

If you try out the therapy a few times, and you don't feel like it is doing anything for you, then it is time to experiment a little bit. Try out a few different methods to see which one seems to provide you the relief that you need. You may find that, by adding just five minutes to your session, you can go from not feeling anything to feeling amazing in no time!

They Didn't Do Their Research

Doing your research about red light therapy is going to make a big difference in the outlook that you have with it, and how much you will be able to use it for. Whether you need some scientific information to figure out if this treatment is effective or not, or you are interested in learning just how this treatment is going to be able to benefit your health, you will find that there is a ton of studies and more on this.

The worst thing about having this lack of research is that people do not know all of the great health benefits they can reap from it. They may have heard about a handful of the health benefits that come with red light therapy, but because they haven't done all of the research, they don't realize that it is possible for them to improve their health condition from it. The more you learn about red light therapy, the more you can see that the treatment can help to benefit anyone who decides to use it.

Even if you have gone through this guidebook and have found that you don't see the condition that you need to have fixed on the list, then this doesn't mean that all hope is lost. It simply means that you need to find the research that points out how great this treatment can be for everyone.

They Are Skeptical About the Process

We have been trained well by the big pharmaceuticals and others who make a lot of money in our world of medicine: We learn that we are supposed to take expensive medications, do expensive surgeries, and sacrifice our health in order to make sure that we can get rid of some disease or illness. It is big business for some companies, but it is not always the best choice for us.

All the information that we have been fed is not in our best interests, but it does make us a skeptic when it comes to some other treatments that work, but don't seem to fit in with what traditional medicine tells us about. This makes it hard, because a lot of people miss out on some of the benefits that come with this kind of treatment, as they don't think that it can work for them, or anyone else.

But there are so many great benefits that come with the use of red light therapy. And it can benefit pretty much anyone who is willing to give it a try. Even if you are a big fan of medicine, surgery and the conventional medical things that we use now, why not give it a try? There are no negative side effects, and just because red light therapy is used, it doesn't mean that you have to completely give up on the other stuff. But why not enhance those a bit? Even if you don't think it works, there are no side effects, and it could be exactly what you are looking for.

They Don't Learn How to Relax All of the Ways

One thing that you need to focus on here is that you need to be able to relax while the red light therapy is doing its job. This may sound like not that big of a deal, but you do want to make sure that you are not tensed up and that the body and the mind is able to relax for the full duration of the therapy, whether it is 15 minutes 20 minutes, or even half an hour or more to get the results.

This may be hard for some people to do. But it is hard for you to get results from any kind of therapy that you try, for any kind of treatment that you try out. Being tense the whole time slows down the process, and you are not going to get the amount of relief that you would like.

There are a few steps that you are able to take that will make it easier to relax. If you need to take a few minutes to do some deep breathing exercises before starting, doing some reading, or even taking a nice bath can help. You may find that a few minutes of meditation will make a difference. You will definitely see a huge difference from doing a session while tensed up and worried, and when you do one after being able to find a method that relaxes you before starting.

Not Choosing the Right Device

The next thing that you need to focus on with this therapy is picking out a device that is going to work for providing you with the needed treatment. You do not want to pick out a device that is not red or infrared technology, or it is not going to do the work that is promised.

This is where you need to be able to do some research ahead of time. There are some high-quality options for devices on the market, but there are also many companies that are trying to jump on the bandwagon which may not offer you the good product that you are looking for. Double check the reviews and the description that comes with the devices to help you make sure that you are going to get the results that you are looking for.

They Don't Put the Light in the Right Spot

This one is a pretty easy one to work through. You just need to make sure that you are setting up the light in a spot where it can be exposed to the problem you want to solve. Probably the hardest situation that comes with this is when you would like to do the light therapy over the whole body, but you are not sure how to get to the whole body. Or, if you want to heal the back, for example, it is going to be most productive if you are able to put it right up against your back.

A bit of research about the right places to put the lights, and knowing where to set it up so you don't have to hold it for the whole time can help. Going back to the example of pain in the back, you may find that laying down on the ground and having the light right to the spot that hurts on your back is going to be the best. If you want to go with the full body, using the fetal position that we talked about in a previous chapter, or setting the lights up so they are above your body and can reach most places can work as well.

Learning how to work with red light therapy is important if you want to see the best results along the way. Luckily, this treatment is going to be safe and effective to use, which is going work wonders for you when you are ready to heal yourself in a natural manner. Watch out for the common mistakes above so that you can be as prepared as possible for getting the full benefits from red light therapy.

Chapter 11: FAQs About Red Light Therapy

It is normal to hear about red light therapy and have some questions. Many people may not have heard about this kind of treatment, and it is a bit different from some of the other therapies and medications that are offered right now. This doesn't make it any less effective to use, but it is important for us to learn about it, and asking questions is one of the best ways to do this. Let's take a look at some of the most common questions people have when it comes to working with red light therapy to help you see if this treatment is the best option for you.

Is Eye Protection Necessary with Red Light Therapy Treatments?

The first question we are going to take a look at here is whether it is necessary to bring in some eye protection when you are working with the red light treatment. As of right now, no patient has reported having issues with their eyes or any eye damage while using light therapy. In fact, doing this kind of treatment has been found to actually improve the eyes and how well they are able to work.

What this means is that, like the other cells of the body, when you keep the eyes open and uncovered, it is likely that you are going to be able to benefit from using this kind of light therapy in your life. The only instance where it may be beneficial to work with eye protection is if you feel that the brightness of the lights is too much for you. But there will not be any negatives if you decide to just turn on the lights without any protection on the eyes.

What is a Wavelength

Since we are talking about light and light therapy, we need to take a look at what a wavelength is all about and why it is important. When we are looking at electromagnetic radiation, like radio waves, the light waves of this treatment are going to travel through space, and they will make a repeating sine wave pattern. The wavelength that we are looking for is just going to be the distance over which the shape of the wave is going to repeat. For example, the red light that is used in this therapy is shorter in wavelength than is near infrared, and far infrared has a wavelength that is even larger.

What Kind of Bulbs Are the Best for the Treatments?

There are a few options that you can choose when it comes to doing your treatments, and knowing which ones are the best for your needs can be important to make sure you actually see the results from your treatments. To start off, incandescent and halogen lights are going to emit about 35 percent of the total power they give out within the range that works in light therapy.

These lights are going to be the best ones for you to work with. Fluorescent lights are different. They emit a bit of ultraviolet light, but it is not likely that they will give any red or near-infrared radiation. This is why we are often going to have some side effects when we expose ourselves to these lights, as compared to red light therapy. In fact, these lights are believed to be a big contributor to a lot of the bad diseases and conditions people throughout the country are dealing with.

Why Are Near-Infrared and Red Lights Better Than Far Infrared Lights?

Red and near-infrared radiation, where the wavelength is going to be somewhere between 500nm to 1500nm, are going to be absorbed by an enzyme that is found within the mitochondria of your cells. We talked about this enzyme earlier, called "cytochrome c oxidase". This is going to result in a greater amount of energy production for that cell as compared to those that haven't been hit with the lights.

Adequate energy is important in the cells because it creates a cell that is healthy. If you are able to get enough of the cells to produce energy in an efficient manner, then it is easier to be healthy. But this is not something that we are going to see with far-infrared technology. This kind of light is not going to be absorbed or used by the enzymes, and this makes it work in a different manner.

When we take a look at far-infrared lights, we see that its wavelength is longer than the others. This one can go through 1500nm to 10,000nm. Because of this difference, the far infrared light is not going to hit the cells and provide them with more energy. Instead, it is going to improve the metabolism of the body by giving a small increase temporarily in the temperature of the body.

The thyroid hormone is responsible for regulating the body temperature, but when this doesn't do its job, raising the body temperature through some other means can help to improve the metabolism. The reason that we may want to work with this is that lowering the overall temperature of the body, even by just one degree, can have a big effect on enzymatic activity. Reduced activity means that the body's metabolic energy production is going to suffer.

What this means is that if the body temperature goes lower than what is seen as ideal, then using an infrared sauna is going to help to restore the function of the enzymes, so that the metabolism is going to be more efficient throughout the body.

Is It Normal to Feel Some Tingling During the Therapy?

Some people have reported feeling a bit of tingling while going through this kind of therapy. According to Dr. Michael Hamblin, this feeling is perfectly normal. It shows up on the skin during the treatment sometimes, and it is basically just the photo-dissociation of the nitric oxide as it starts to separate from the cytochrome c oxidase enzyme in the cell. This means that the light therapy is doing exactly what it promised, and you will start seeing the results in no time.

How Does Pulsed Red Light Therapy Work?

Another thing that you may consider when you are working with red light therapy is the idea of pulsed light therapy. This one is going to be pretty much the same, but instead of just having the light stay steady on the part of the body that you are trying to heal, you are going to have the light blink on and off at regular intervals during the therapy.

The idea of pulsed red light therapy is just going to be flickering on and off of the red light at a specific frequency for the pulses. This therapy is going to affect the cells in the same way as the traditional continuous wave therapy that we have talked about in this guidebook, and it does this by enhancing the ATP production within the mitochondria of the cell.

But some people are interested in seeing if the pulsed light therapy will be any different, or more or less effective than traditional therapy. When you are comparing these, there will be some conflicting evidence. There are some studies that are going to indicate that the pulsing light is the most effective, and there are some s that say that the continuous light is the best.

One of the studies that were recently done to compare pulsed therapy to regular therapy was done by Dr. Michael Hamblin. He was able to write an extensive review of these therapies and took the time to look at the effects of many different frequencies to see what would work the best, and whether they were pulsed or not.

Basically, what was found in this review is that both of these therapies work. The important thing is that you use the red light, not whether it is pulsed or not. You are going to get the benefits in any case. If you do choose to work with the pulsed therapy, make sure that your frequency is slow and steady, rather than too fast. When you let the light go too fast, it is just going to confuse the cells and will make you lose the benefits. Most patients who decide to go with the pulsed therapy find that doing between 10HZ and 100HZ is perfect to get started.

The choice to go with pulsed light is going to be completely up to you. You need to choose whether you are more comfortable with the steady light or the pulsed light, and which one is giving you the most benefits. Listening to your body and experimenting a bit along the way is the best choice, no matter how you use the red light therapy.

It is normal to have a lot of questions when it comes to working with red light therapy, no matter what kind of method you want to go with, or what condition you want to heal. Make sure to read through this information and ask any questions that you have to ensure that you fully understand all of the ways that this therapy is able to help you.

Chapter 12: Methods to Use to Accelerate Your Healing with Light Therapy

Now that we know a bit more about red light therapy and all of the things that you are able to do with it, it is time to delve a bit more into some of the things that you are able to do in order to see this therapy really come to life and do a lot for you.

While the red light therapy is going to be powerful on its own, you will find that there are a few actions that you are able to take to enhance it further. These actions are often simple, but they are going to propel you along on this journey and will make results faster and more efficient. Some of the steps that you can use in order to get the most out of the red light therapy include:

Do Two Sessions a Day

You can certainly choose to just work with one session a day if you would like, but many times, people find that they are going to get the most out of their treatment when they are able to do two or even three sessions during the day. The trick here is to experiment and see what is going to work the best for you.

When you choose to do the light therapy more than once a day, you are really working on healing the cells and keeping all of that nitric acid out of the body. And you are going to be amazed at the difference this makes. You will feel like there is more energy inside of you when it is time to start the morning, and it can be a nice way to turn the body down after a long day of working and putting aside all of your other obligations for the day.

Of course, if you find that only one treatment is able to do the work that you need, or you just find that it is difficult to fit the sessions in more than once, then it is fine to stick with that number of sessions for your needs. But many patients who use this therapy and see the best results with it are going to really like working with the red light at least a few times a day.

Get Plenty of Sleep

The next thing that we need to focus on here is the idea of getting yourself plenty of sleep on a regular basis. When you are short on sleep, you are not giving your body the time that it needs to replenish itself or clean out some of the toxins that plague it. Even if you are working with the red light therapy, if you are not taking in enough sleep on a regular basis, then the body is not going to be able to clear itself out, and you are not going to feel better.

But getting enough sleep on a regular basis can be a struggle for many people. Learning how to take care of yourself, getting off the phone, and reducing your levels of stress are all necessary if you would like to get sleep at night. But some of the things that you are able to do to help you get to sleep fast and stay asleep all night includes:

1. Keep work at work: If you often bring your work home with you, then it is going to be hard for you to really learn how to get to bed on time. This kind of lifestyle often means that you are stressed, and won't be able to turn your mind off when it is time to go to bed.

2. Turn off electronics before bed: If possible, turn off all electronics about an hour before going to bed. This helps to detoxify the brain from the light emitted from the computer, phone, and more so that it can relax. Consider

reading, writing, or starting your bedtime routine during this time instead.

3. Make a list of the things you need to do the next day: It is hard to get to sleep at night if you have a million thoughts and things to remember running through your brain. Before you head to bed, make a list of the things that you want to get done, so you no longer have to worry about remembering them later on.

4. Be more active during the day: If you are sitting at a desk all day, or not doing much, then it may be hard to keep up your activity levels. Instead of letting that happen, you need to find ways to be more active so that your brain is ready to go to sleep. Whether that means getting up and moving more, or starting a workout routine, you have to find the method of activity that works the best for you.

5. Start a nighttime routine: Having a routine is a good way to tell your brain that it is time to

turn off and go to bed. And starting this a while before you hit the hay is going to make a world of difference as well. You can make it as long, as short, as easy, or as complicated as you would like. Just stick with the same routine each day.

6. Turn off the lights: Sleeping in the dark is usually the best. You will find that this helps to signal to the brain that it is time to go to sleep. Find any of the lights that are in the room that may be keeping you awake at night and figure out how to turn them off or get rid of them.

7. No television in the bedroom: There are a lot of people who like to fall asleep with a TV in their room. They think that this helps them to fall asleep at night. While you may be able to get to sleep with the noise and the light of the television going, your sleep is not going to be very deep. Turn it off or get it out of the

room, and see what a difference it is able to make for you.

8. Listen to some quiet and soft music if needed: Some people find that either the noises outside their windows are too loud, or they just have trouble with the quiet. If this is the case for you, do not let it be an excuse to go out and grab the television. Instead, turn on some soft classical music or some music to the sounds of nature, and let that be what helps to lull you to sleep at night.

Getting enough sleep is going to be critical if you would like to really see the benefits that come with red light therapy. It is hard to do this, but putting yourself first, and learning when to say no to other obligations and temptations can help to make it a bit easier.

Eat Lots of Healthy Foods

To help your cells to function well, and if you want to get the most out of the red light therapy, then you need to be more aware of the foods that you are consuming. You do not want to do the red light therapy and then go fill up on brownies and ice cream the whole time. Instead, filling the body up with foods that are healthy and will give the body the nutrition it needs to get healthier and to do the necessary repairs, is going to be critical.

This brings up the question of how you are supposed to eat in a healthy manner.
You do not need to follow a strict diet or go on something that is hard to follow. If you want to lose more weight while doing the treatment, that is fine, but by eating foods that are good for you, and made with real ingredients rather than processed ingredients, then you are going to see better results as well.

So, to make sure that you are eating foods that are going to help fill you up and will make sure that you are getting the nutrition that you need, think about foods in their natural states. Eating lots of fresh fruits and vegetables, lean sources of meat and protein, using healthy oils for cooking, good dairy products with no added sugars, and whole grain carbohydrates will do the trick. Learn how to do the right portion sizes, and how to listen to your body when it is hungry or not, and you will start to see results with your health as well.

Learn How to Get Rid of the Junk

While it may be fine to have a bit of junk food on occasion when you crave something sweet, most of us enjoy way too many sweets and junk food that we do not need. We take in lots of carbohydrates, sugars, baked goods, sodas and juices, and so much more. And this ends up being really bad for us overall.

If you want to be able to reduce the problems that you have with your cells and many diseases, you need to help the red light treatment out a bit by cutting out some of the junk. Limit yourself to just a bit of those on occasion, rather than making it a staple in your diet plan. This can be hard, and you may need to go through a bit of a detoxification to make it happen. But if you are able to stick with this, you are going to see some major changes in your health.

Drink Lots of Water

You will want to make sure that you are getting all of the toxins out of your body during this treatment, while also staying hydrated and making sure that your organs and all parts of your body are going to work well. Too many times, we are too busy with our days, or be drinking coffee, pop, and other drinks, and we do not make sure that we are going to be able to give the body the optimal hydration that we need from water.

It should be your goal to take in a minimum of eight to ten glasses of water a day. If you are still thirsty after that, do exercise, or are dealing with a day that is really hot, then try to drink more. This is going to help you to get as much out of the red light therapy as possible, and even a little bit extra water in your day will be enough to help you to feel better too.

Try to Avoid Stress (As Much as Possible)

If you read this tip and rolled your eyes, then you are not alone. It seems like there is always more than enough stress and stressful situations to go around in our modern world, and learning how to avoid that stress, or at least limit it as much as possible, can seem like an impossible task to complete. But the more that you are able to reduce and eliminate the stress in your body, the healthier you are going to be overall.

There are a number of things that you are able to do in order to limit the amount of stress that you already feel in your life. Some of the best suggestions include:

1. Learn how to say no: It is common for people to fall into the habit of saying yes when someone makes a request to them. Don't feel bad if you are already too busy and are not able to help out. Learn when you can take on more, and when you just can't handle it.

2. Learn meditation: Even a few minutes while you work on the light therapy can help to relax your mind, and you will feel the stress levels start to melt away until you are no longer able to feel them.

3. Take a warm bath. This will help you to calm the mind, and could help to spur the cells on to more energy and faster healing.

4. Spend time with friends: It is easy, with all the things we need to get done during the day, to be too busy to slow down and concentrate on the connections that we need. Slow down a bit and learn how to make more connections, spend more time, and be closer with your friends and family.

5. Exercise: A bit of exercise is going to do wonders for detoxing the body and helping you to get even more results overall.

6. Do something that you enjoy: You will find that taking even a small amount of time each day to do something that you love can help to reduce the amount of stress that you are going to feel.

Dealing with stress is never a good thing when it comes to your overall health, and it is best if you are able to find some methods that will reduce this. Following the steps above, and learning what works the best for you will ensure that your stress levels are kept down to a minimum.

There are already a lot of great benefits that come with doing some light therapy in your life. But when you add in the examples and suggestions that we talked about in this chapter, you will find that it is so much easier to see the healing and the good health that you want, all from just doing a bit of red light therapy treatment in the day.

Chapter 13: Tips to Get the Most Out of Your Red Light Therapy

At this point, we have spent a lot of time learning about red light therapy and all of the neat things it is able to do for your health. We spent time looking at the different health benefits that come with this therapy, the different methods that you can use to make sure that the red light ends up on the right part of your body to do their work, and so much more.

Now that we have some of that information out of the way, it is time to look at a few tips that you can follow in order to get the most out of this therapy option. While you are sure to see some great results just by putting the light on you and leaving it there alone for a few times a day, there are a few tips and suggestions that you can follow that will help you to really get the most out of each and every session you do. Some of the tips that you may find useful with red light therapy treatments include:

1. Make sure that the light box that you use provides you with a full spectrum of bright white light, while also ensuring that it is able to block all of the ultraviolet lights. It is best if it is able to filter out 99 percent of these rays because they are seen as really harmful to your body.

2. Position the box so that it is at eye level or higher. The position, as well as the distance of your light box in connection with your eyes, is going to make a difference. You want to try and get this light box to mimic what happens when you are outside in the sun.

3. Place the box so that it ends up a few feet from your eyes. It is best to put it around two feet from the eyes at the time of use. Of course, if you already know that the light in your box is a bit weaker, then you will want to move it closer. This advice is going to work the best if your box is a 10,000 Lux box.

Adjust the distance based on what your box is to this amount.

4. Keep the light box so that it is more at an angle than straight on. You may find that having it at 10 or 2 degrees is the best position to get the benefits. It is not usually recommended for you to place the light right in your eye frame or right on the problem you are trying to fix. It is best to position it so that the light falls 45 degrees to the left or the right from the middle point of your eyes.

5. Go with a box that is about 10,000 Lux. You do not want to work with a normal lamp, because you will not get the red light from this. The 10,000 Lux will make it strong enough so that you are going to be able to get the benefits, and in the meantime without having to worry about it being too strong or too weak for you to use.

6. Be consistent with the use of the box: It is best for you to use the box on a regular basis

to get the best results. If you only use it occasionally when you think about it, or when someone else reminds you about it, then this is not a good thing. You are going to end up missing out on some of the cool things that can happen with regular use of the red light therapy, and you are not going to be as impressed with the results that you are able to get.

7. If you are taking some medications at the time, talk to your doctor about using light therapy. This is often not going to be too big of a problem, but there are some medications that may not react the way that you would like when the red light is put on them. It could be that the medication makes your skin more sensitive to light and that can change up the skin in a manner that looks like a rash or sunburn. You can talk to your doctor to see if this is a problem for you or not.

8. Pick a time frame that works the best for you: You have to be able to pick the times that work the best for you. Whether you are picking between morning and evening, or both, or you are deciding between five minutes or twenty minutes, you need to go with a time frame that is going to work the best for your schedule, time, and what you feel the most comfortable with doing.

9. Pick out a good body position as well. You need to be able to pick a good position to do the light therapy in. Most of the time, it is recommended that you do light therapy while lying down. But if you find that standing up or sitting down is the best option for you, then go ahead and work with that option. The point here is that you need to pick the position that makes you the most comfortable, and will help you to relax completely. If you are not able to relax and get comfortable with the light therapy, then it is

129

going to be hard to get the full benefits when you start your red light therapy.

10. Monitor the condition or your mood after the red light therapy to see if it is working. Even just a few minutes with the therapy is going to be enough to improve your mood. You may notice it right after you are done with the therapy. Other times, it may be a day or two after the therapy when you start to notice a change. You will feel happier, have less anxiety, and have more energy overall.

11. Combine this therapy with some other approaches that we have talked about in this guidebook to give yourself the best results possible. Adding in some other therapies like the ones that we talked about above will help you to really get the benefits of red light therapy.

Working with red light therapy is going to be one of the best things that you are going to be able to do for your overall health, whether you are trying to lose weight, alleviate your pain, help with cell repair, improve your memory, or so much more. Learning how this therapy works, and using some of the tips above for this red light therapy is going to make a big difference in the way that you feel.

Unlike some of the medications you may have taken in the past, or that your doctor and others have talked about getting you on in the future, you will be able to work with red light therapy and not have to worry about any of its negative side effects. You will get the benefits of enjoying good health and less pain, among a lot of other benefits, while doing it in a manner that is natural for you. Think of how great you are going to feel if you can just start using some red light therapy on a consistent basis, with the tips that we discussed in this chapter!

Conclusion

Thanks for making it through to the end of *Red Light Therapy*! Let's hope it was informative and able to provide you with all of the tools you need to achieve your goals, whatever they may be.

The next step is to decide when you would like to use red light therapy. No matter what kind of condition you are dealing with, or how much you need to repair your body, you will find that you are able to benefit when you use red light therapy, whether it is from a disease or even stress and pain! This guidebook will spend some time talking about red light therapy in order to show you how you will be able to get the most benefits from its usage.

Whether you are interested in the science of this therapy, or you are more interested in learning the steps that you need to get the most out of the red light therapy (such as how to start your own session), this guidebook is going to spend some time talking about everything that is needed with this kind of therapy plan.

When you are ready to use red light therapy to boost your overall health, or you are mainly interested in learning more about this treatment option before you get started, make sure to check out this guidebook first.

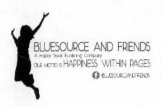

BLUESOURCE AND FRIENDS
A Happy Book Publishing Company
OUR MOTTO IS HAPPINESS WITHIN PAGES
/BLUESOURCEANDFRIENDS

Connect with us on our Facebook page

www.facebook.com/bluesourceandfriends and stay

tuned to our latest book promotions and free

giveaways.